FRENCH CHIC

50 French Style & Beauty 'Secrets'

Thank You!

I wanted to start off by just saying thank you for choosing to read one of my books. I know there are millions of other books out there and how valuable your time is so I am extremely thankful that you took the time out of your day to read my book.

I wanted to also quickly explain to you that you are actually getting an extra book from me within this one book you purchased. I have included practically ALL of my books that I have available on Amazon at no additional cost to you. I wanted to give you all of these bonus books as my way of saying thank you!

BON CHIC, BON GENRE!

Secret #1 Good Style, Good Attitude

Bon chic, bon genre' is an expression used in France to refer to a stylish subculture, meaning 'Good Style=Good Attitude.' <u>The better you dress the better you feel.</u> (The expression can also be shortened as 'BCBG' which is also known as the fashion company BCBG Max Azria.) French style is to embody elegance, polish, and minimalism. Parisian style also can be defined as 'effortless', and in no way over-studied. In case you're aware of a Parisian woman in Paris, you'll see her shoes are manufactured from exceptional leather, her jumper is of cashmere, and her shirt is spun silk. French style is to be conscious of quality, and not so much on quantity, while mixing and matching. It is about starting out with the right pieces that you can mix and match to wear anywhere. And, not obsessing about it. Have the poise to feel elegant yet slightly off beat, polished but not glitzy, and self-confident enough to understand that the true meaning of chic is very individual.

It's about the entire outfit running in unison as opposed to tossing on random garments like a train wreck after which leaving the house. She makes an attempt no matter how she feels. Parisians know how to ensemble outfits in a manner which makes you agree that every piece is remarkable.

They don't dress down, and they don't own hoodies, or visit the cafe in yoga pants. Parisians don't second guess their fashion picks or ask for style critiques, they dress for themselves.

Secret #2 Mix & Match Without Many Embellishments

The first rule of French style is the focus on unique shapes and patterns without many embellishments. It is about looking natural, and having the allure of life.

Secret #3 Edit Your Wardrobe

Perhaps, since because most Paris apartments don't provide an extensive amount of space in the closet, Parisian style is very well edited to consist of the most practical pieces to work collectively from head to toe. Every element of the outfit is prepared to work as an entire. In Paris, you won't see ladies strolling around in lumpy parkas which hit their hip at the incorrect location and does not do anything for the rest of their outfit- it's a completely meticulous way that every form or layer provides directly to create the right silhouette. French splendor has a less is more mindset that is not self-conscious. That means no long, garish fake fingernails, no heavy powdery makeup, no over waxed eyebrows, no over bleached yellow blonde hair, and no crispy hair gel, and no fake orange sun tan skin. In order for you to achieve 'French Chic' you wouldn't need to put on something tight, like a body con dress, or something that shows an excessive amount of skin.

As an alternative, go for looser apparel, with maybe a flash of shoulder or ankle, and a waft of your preferred French fragrance ex. Chanel No. 5. Show a little skin, in surprising ways, like your back, or a glimpse the shoulders. What you do see in terms of 'French Chic' beauty are plenty of gorgeous brunettes with simple, stylishly undone hair, natural eyebrows, minimal appearing makeup with a "no makeup" feel, smoldering kohl lined eyes, natural lip color and (or) a bold crimson lip stain all creating the facade of better than natural, but still very approachable, confident, and unfussed.

Secret #4 Posture Matters

Here is the cheapest and easiest French Chic beauty secret that you can steal, stand straight! There is not a better way to show off self-confidence in your appearance than having perfect, erect posture and presenting yourself with pride.

Secret #5 No Brand Flashing!

Notably, despite the fact that Louis Vuitton is a French company. You won't see many local Parisian women carrying LV baggage in Paris. So, no brand flashing, while embracing French style. The iconic French woman is robust, and is visible in lots of advertisements. She is the woman who cuts her hair herself. She is subtle, sexy, with a combination of nonchalant, self-assurance, mystery, and effortlessness. To Parisian ladies, going out is just a matter of dressing up a bit.

Secret #6 Own Your Femininity

They go out of the house to look presentable, and they don't try too hard. French style is also about owning your femininity. This does not suggest that you constantly need to wear a dress or a skirt. It just means to embrace your femininity every day.

Ensure that your hair is properly conditioned and moisturized. Irrespective of what the style your hair is in, because it will look amazing due to you taking great care of it. Make sure your nails are manicured, neat, and shiny.

STARTING WITH THE BASICS

Secret #7 Neutrals Rule

Neutrals are the key palette when it comes to French style. Parisian ladies tend to not wear a variety of colors. That is, barely any. If they do wear it, it's in accessories like their scarves, jewelry, shoes, luggage, etc. You recognize stuff like that. The brightest they get is after they put on some ivory or white, with perhaps a pop a burgundy. In any other case, their color palette is pretty miserable to the general public. Here is the Parisian color palette:

Black

Grey

Navy

Brown

White

Burgundy

Black is one the primary colors in Parisian wardrobes (a lot like the Big Apple, which is probably why they may be so frequently as compared to each other.) Grey is the runner-up, after which they use dark blue or brown as a color for leather-based fashions. Fun, right? You can't live without a little frivolity,

Incorporate color and print into your accessories (although not all at once) Go for a fire engine red lipstick, a pair of leopard print pumps with a sculpted heel, or an easy Hermès tooth bracelet in your favorite color that pops.

Secret #8 The Basics

When choosing to dress 'French Chic' you'll want to start with the following basics:

A crisp white blouse (A white button down is a vital building block in anyone's closet, at least for the French. Opt for a linen or brushed cotton shirt in the smallest size you can find, leave the tails half and simply roll up the sleeves. Instant French-chic, and in and clothes you can move in. The same white shirt also does double duty as an easy breezy cover-up by the pool when the summer rolls around. And let's face it; Who wouldn't want the best of both worlds?)

A black skirt-ideally knee length or A-line which is the most flattering

Fitted suit jacket, blazer (Look for structured shoulders, and keep away from sweatshirts or something with a noisy label.)

A properly cut feminine leather-based jacket or biker jacket

T-shirts (make sure they consist of some with stripes-the uber chic long sleeve striped top is effortlessly cool, and will preserve your heat on cool Paris nights. Instead of opting for the classic black and white stripe layout you could always go for striped shirts with a special color like pink or even a vibrant blue.)

Tank tops

Lightweight cashmere cardigans (they don't itch and are pretty versatile-they also go along with skirts and pants, and they're light enough to wear in the spring and summer months. Tie-front cardigans are ok, simply ensure your wear a white or colored camisole below them.)

An excellent, nicely fitting pair of dark denim or stretch denim (you'll be able to dress them up or down-Denim is a simple and essential way to stay cool and modern in any season. The proper pair of cropped denim that fits your frame is understatedly sexy, while remaining sophisticated. Darker wash denim tends to appear more luxe and dressier than lighter wash denims.)

A couple of properly fitting black pants- immediately creates a refined and assured look.

A pair of elegant comfy shoes in a solid color

A light trench coat in a neutral color (The trench coat has no question formed an integral part of the Parisian wardrobe, it has great use and has the effortless ability to be worn to any weather condition. Trench coats, pea coats, female leather jackets, and cropped or outfitted blazers all give the appearance of chic without being fussy.)

An awesome quality bag (Go for a luxe, quilted handbag, with rich fabric, and lustrous hardware-A Chanel purse, in particular the vintage 2.55, consists of these types of details in a single pretty package deal. In case you aren't inclined to break the bank for this well-known bag, use the simple bone shape when selecting one most suitable for your lifestyle. A square or square formed shoulder bag with glossy hardware and polished leather will add that Parisian finishing flair you're seeking out.)

Scarves in all colors, styles, and sizes (Keep reading to discover ways to tie them-Smart add-ons like a neck scarf give a touch of ladylike appeal to any outfit. It can be a fascinating accent that lets you play with some color, pattern, and print in a small way that won't overpower the rest of your outfit. Choose scarves with the intention to pop in opposition to your minimalist look for a true statement.)

Black tights, or sheer natural toned stockings (not leggings)

The proper undies (comfortable and preferably attractive if that's feasible)

Sunglasses (Oversized sunglasses are always super chic-in the event that they suit your face shape, it can be an easy way to work an accessory into your outfit in case you are not a fan of the neck or headscarf. A tortoise shell print is vintage inspired, especially if worn in cat eye form. Round formed sun shades generally match a variety of face shapes, and a cat eye design is flirty and feminine, defining the very essence of the city of Paris.)

Remember that it's not always what you wear, but how you wear it. Dress casual, yet simple and fashionable, no disheveled sweats or oversized items of apparel. Same goes for something that's too tight. Fitted doesn't mean tight. Don't wear anything tacky or over the top. Moderation applies to garments and add-ons too. A tailored cut equals a slimmer silhouette. Parisian women also don't over accessorize. As Coco Chanel once said, "Before you leave the house, look in the mirror and remove one accessory."

LESS IS MORE

The French approach hair and beauty much like their approach to getting dressed: less is more. In European culture, skin care is a primary task. They keep their skin hydrated, and take the time to shop around for great skin care products at a number of pharmacies and cosmetic stores at the local Galleries Lafayette.

Secret #9 Invest In Good Skin Care

A Parisian typically does not attempt to cover up their skin to make for the appearance of perfection. If they have acne, they have acne. French women are taught from a younger age that taking great care of your skin which is a crucial component for long term beauty. Every year a dermatologist visit is vital, and lots of French women use different creams and cleansers for day vs. night. Ex. Vitamin C creams, Retin-A, and Argan Oil. It is also not unusual in French culture to make personal body scrubs with oil and sea salt.

Secret #10 Facial Masks

Masks are great to balance, brighten, and hydrate the skin. Masks are usually included in the beauty routine once or twice a week to feed the skin and hair. Homemade masks are typically made from egg yolks, and are kept on for 20 minutes and washed with vinegar water.

Secret #11 Intensive Skin Care Creams

The French reach for skin care products, such as skin creams, over cosmetics. They rather have a healthy and super clear complexion; and they keep it simple by moisturizing with natural oils to nourish the skin and hair.

Secret #12 Hydration Is Important

Drinking a glass of water is very important, especially before bed, and the first thing in the morning. Water is the Parisian woman's special secret-for health, skin, and beauty. Water flushes toxins and controls weight.

Secret #13 Choose Water Over Snacks

Reaching for the snack cupboard when feeling a bit puckish, instead of drinking a glass of water is bad habit that we need to break. When your body needs water, sometimes it can be mistaken as hunger pains. French women are great a drinking lots of water. The next time your craving a snack, think twice and give this French secret a try, and your hunger pains will almost disappear instantly.

Secret #14 Makeup

If you chose to wear makeup: in essence, you'll want to go for natural look that emphasizes your natural beauty, rather than looking like you have loads of makeup on. Foundation is key. Choosing the right foundation color should be an easy task, just match according to the shade of your palm. Take your foundation, and apply it to your face (One pump on average should cover your entire face.) Start blending outwards with a beauty sponge or foundation brush to get an airbrushed natural effect. Opt for a black kohl liner and smudge outwards for a smoky effect. When focusing on the lips, go for neutral lip balm. Finish with the look with a mild sweep of mascara- often one coat for daytime, and two for night time.

Secret #15 Say Yes to a Red Lip

Red lipstick is style accessory. When you wear it, apply neutral makeup, because the lipstick makes the declaration. Try a matte scarlet or crimson lipstick.

Secret #16 Don't Wash Your Hair

Okay, wash your hair, but not every day. Too much washing can strip your hair of its natural oils. For the French lady, it's all about texture. They generally tend to pull away from American hair tendencies, such as blow-outs, and hair straightening. It's the bed-head, lived in look you'll notice around Paris. When caring for your hair, finger-combing is best to achieve the undone French hair look. Finger-combing creates the perfect amount of tousle and texture, which can be enhanced with a bit of sea salt spray. Another hair styling choice is a pixie-cut, it's low on upkeep is a way to attain understated sophistication.

Secret #17 Mix Self Tanner with Daily Moisturizer to Cover Dark Spots

It can sometimes be a challenge to preserve a clear complexion. If you have a few dark spots that you want to cover while still being French chic, mix a pea-sized amount of self-tanner into your daily moisturizer. You may additionally include a small amount into your body cream.

Secret #18 Your Nail Polish Should Stay Cold

Maintain your favorite polishes in the refrigerator; by keeping them chilled it's going to last a lot longer and go on much more smoothly.

Secret #19 Use an Eye Mask as an Eye Lash Curler

When I'm on an airplane and ready to sleep, I slide on my eye mask so that it bends my eyelashes upwards. It works like an eyelash curler, and when I wake up, my eyes look more awake and open. But, you don't have to get on a plane for this trick to work.

Secret #20 Make Your Purse Smell Good

Sprits a cotton handkerchief with your favorite fragrance and keep it in your purse. The contents will smell amazing, on every occasion that you decide to open your bag.

Secret #21 Get the Glow

French women aren't afraid to turn on the cold water near the end of a shower to get one's circulation going. Using warm water to open the pores and then cold water to close them is a part of their beauty routine. The sudden change in temperature boosts blood circulation to the skin, and makes the skin glow.

Secret #22 Workout Outdoors

The French don't prefer to workout indoors. You won't see many Parisians indoors, working out at a gym. They choose to exercise via water cardio instructions, aqua gymnasium, and a different variety of fun activities. They also practice 'invisible workouts.' Which is adding a bits of exercising to your daily routine, some examples are deciding to park the car farther from the grocery store entrance or taking the stairs instead of the elevator.

Secret #23 Facial Massages

Facial Massages are the norm, and help even out skin tone. Getting a good massage can help you feel refreshed. You can choose to have very own facial massage by simply winking the eyes, doing various facial exercises, and massaging your cheeks.

Secret #24 Home Remedies Are The Best

The market for beauty products is over abundant with options; sometimes it can be difficult to find exactly what's best for your skin. Clean your face every night before going to bed, and apply the following strawberry-honey mix mask recipe for the face. Rinse your hair with cold water and an added tablespoon of vinegar or lemon juice for added shine before moisturizing.

Strawberry-Honey Mask Ingredients:

6 fresh Destemmed Strawberries

2 Tablespoons of Organic Honey

2/4 Fresh Lemon Juice From Wedge

Secret #25 Anti-aging

Anti-aging is seen from within. Parisians don't stress, and aren't afraid of aging. They believe in looking natural, with the help of oils, honey, shea butter, and extracts. Aging is an attitude, you can look great at any age! Homemade juices are amazing for anti-aging.

Secret #26 Avoid Too Much Exfoliation

Try to avoid too much exfoliation on the skin. Exfoliating once or twice a week with a natural face scrub can be beneficial, and will help soothe, replenish, and soften the skin. Remember to always exfoliate with care.

Secret #27 Wine

Wine is a top French beauty secret. It is packed with antioxidants, and is great for your skin and body. (Moderation is key.)

Secret #28 Never Go To Bed With Makeup Still On

The French rarely wear makeup, but when they do, they don't ever go to bed with their makeup left on. Going to bed with makeup on can age skin. So, remember to wash your face with a good makeup remover or cleanser before going to sleep.

Secret #29 Never Eat Processed Foods

Avoid processed foods as much as possible. Try to eat 'whole foods' that don't come from a box, can, or fast food restaurant. An occasional treat is fine. Quality, not quantity.

FIND A BALANCE

Secret #30 Balance

When the summertime comes along, all the color is on my toes! So, when my pedicures get colorful, my manicure stays neutral. Find a balance.

Secret #31 Use Thermal Water Spray

French ladies swear by thermal water spray, it gets rid of harmful chemicals on your face & neck areas from use of tap water. By using thermal water spray you'll soften and refresh your skin. It also allows for better penetration of your favorite toners, creams etc. Wake up your skin with this great French beauty secret.

Secret #32 No Staring at the sun

Another great French beauty secret is to avoid direct sun exposure. Vitamin D is good for the skin, but the direct exposure from the sun is not.

Secret #33 Wear Perfume

Each morning, choose your perfume for the day, depending on how you feel, the weather, or what you decide to wear. Before getting dressed, spritz on your chosen perfume for a soft lingering fragrance that makes a subtle statement.

Secret #34 Don't Touch Your Face

Try not to touch your face, and make sure to wash your hands every chance you get! When traveling around Paris, your hands accumulate dirt and bacteria quickly. Touchng your face, can cause breakouts. In, Paris this is a big no-no!

Secret #35 Don't Be Afraid To Go To Extremes

Always moisturize skin properly, and avoid sun exposure. Try using a higher SPF protectors, such as SPF 50+ and wear a hat, or carry an umbrella. It might be extreme, but it's the best way to care for the skin, and keeping a healthier youthful appearance.

Secret #36 Find Your Beauty Staples-And Stick With Them

When you find a favorite beauty product or staple, be sure to stick with it. Finding something that works for you or your skin is great!

PLUS SECRETS DE BEAUTE

Secret #37 Spend Time Away From Your Hairbrush

The French don't use hair brushes often. So ditch the hairbrush and try using your fingers to 'finger comb' instead.

Secret #38 Living By The Pleasure Principle

The pleasure principle is simple. Your beauty routine should make you feel good and make you look good. Enjoy life, smile, and be happy.

Secret #39 Makeup Remover

Harsh facial cleansers are not a big no, no! Instead, use sweet almond oil as a gentle cleanser and moisturizer to remove any makeup residue

Secret #40 Find Multiple Ways To Use Your Favorite Product

My favorite beauty product at the moment is Argan oil. I apply it to ends of my hair to the root, before I decide to shampoo. During winter months, my skin tends to be a little drier, so I like to incorporate it into my facial cream. It works so well, as a moisturizer!

Secret #41 Heritage

French women learn most of their beauty secrets from relatives starting at a young age. Mothers, and grandmothers pass down their beauty secrets to their children for great looking skin and faces.

Secret #42 Tanning Is A No

French women know the dangers of sun bathing too long. They rather use bottled tan rather than actually getting a tan itself. Make sure to wear SPF whenever you go out, or try to include it in your daily moisturizer. Protect your skin as much as possible.

Secret #43 Walk For 20-Minutes After Every Meal

Walking for 20-minutes after every meal can be beneficial because it decreases your sugar spike in your system. Doing so can also improve your mood, burn calories, and clear your mind. It's one of the ways the French stay slim, and is also why they have better overall health and skin.

Secret #44 Stick To A Mediterranean Diet

A Mediterranean consists of lots of vegetables, fresh fruit, wholegrain cereal, olive oil, nuts, poultry and fish. Try to eliminate red meat, butter, and animal fat. It helps the skin appear flawless, and has great health benefits.

Secret #45 Choose A Non-Impact Workout

You can cut running out of you exercising routine, and not feel bad about it. Running against the concrete can have a shocking effect on your body. The constant up and down motion can cause loosing of facial ligaments and cause sagging of the cheeks and jaw. Instead, try lower-impact exercises, which are popular in France, such as yoga or pilates.

Secret #46 Facials Are Not A Luxury, But An Essential

Beauty facials aren't viewed as a luxury, but for French women it is considered a necessity in their skin car routine. Facials increase blood flow circulation, and allows for the skin to renew itself from dead skin cells. Facials also promote radiant skin.

Secret #47 Make Sleep Your Priority

The benefits of getting eight hours of sleep are endless. The French pay a lot of attention to the boudoir. They make sleep a priority and like to invest in the most luxurious bedding and pillows. Silk sheets will cause less friction on your face, and will decrease your chances of developing wrinkles over time.

Secret #48 Try Highlighting Instead Of Contouring

The beauty philosophy in France is to accept who you are. They keep it simple, so contouring is not much of a norm. Try 'Strobing' or highlighting instead.

Secret #49 Go For A Bun-And Make It Messy

The Messy-Bun is a French must-have. Start with tousled wavy hair and finger comb up, then tie with a band. There you go, a messy-bun.

Secret #50 Accept Physical Imperfections And Embrace Them

The strength in French women lies in their uniqueness. Embrace your imperfections, we are all meant to standout. Individuality is beautiful.

Thanks for reading this book, I hope you found these style and beauty secrets helpful. Feel free to adopt them into your daily routine.

EPSOM SALT

150 Extraordinary Natural Remedies, Uses, and
Benefits for Your Health, Body, Beauty, & Home

Contents

WHAT IS EPSOM SALT?

Epsom Salt was discovered hundreds of years ago (in 1618) in a water spring in Epsom, a village in Surrey (England) after a farmer discovered that although his cows were unhappy with the bitter taste of spring water which they drunk, they were healed of their rashes and scratches. The good news about this miracle product soon spread and it began to be prepared by boiling down spring water, which contained porous chalk material from North Downs (UK) combined with non-porous clay silt from London. This combination resulted in the creation of a crystal like mineral containing magnesium and sulfur which is today referred to as the Epsom Salt.

Epsom salt is also known as magnesium sulfate and is considered as a pure, naturally occurring mineral compound with some amazing healing and beautifying properties.

Since the mineral is quick to absorb water and bacteria, it was commonly used by doctors all over the world to sanitize medical tools and instruments.

Epsom Salt is also included in the World Health Organization's Model List of Essential Medicines (owing to its numerous uses).

The common society still uses it as a bath salt, and it is a favorite with athletes aspiring to relieve themselves from muscle aches and pains.

As you read through the book, you will get to understand the various uses of Epsom Salt which make it much more than just an added luxury in your bath salt.

Besides its ability to heal the body from many physical ailments and health conditions, Epsom Salt also boasts of several household, beautifying, detoxifying, and gardening related benefits.

THINGS TO REMEMBER BEFORE GETTING STARTED

Some people may get a reaction from magnesium – it may lead to a stomach upset or other complications if consumed in large, unsafe amounts. Always consult a doctor if you suspect that you are unwell.

Consult with a qualified medical practitioner and/or doctor before using Epsom Salt and the recipes provided in this book. In case you suffer from any medical condition, allergies, or are pregnant. Readers who fail to consult with appropriate health authorities assume and are responsible for the risk of any injuries. The respective authors and publisher are not liable.

This book is meant for informational purposes only. It is NOT intended to be used as a medical source. This book is NOT meant to be a substitute for medical advice. This book is NOT meant to be taken over any advice provided by your doctor or medical professional. This health book is NOT intended to be used for diagnosing or treating a problem or disease. The natural health information have NOT been evaluated by any statutory or professional body and are not intended to diagnose, treat, cure, or prevent any disease.

Never go overboard with Epsom Salt and use only the recommended dose as and when needed.

Never let your pets consume Epsom Salt.

Always ensure that the type of Epsom Salt you are using contains magnesium sulfate as its main ingredient.

Never use Epsom Salt on children below six years of age.

Before you get started with Epsom Salt, use wisely and with caution, especially if you are using it for healthcare.

If you are a diabetic or suffer from dry, cracked or fragile skin, use gentle foot soaks instead of a full body soak.

If you are using all the precautions mentioned above, nothing can be as miraculous as Epsom Salt. This book covers 150 amazing uses of Epsom Salt. These uses have been divided into various categories but have been numbered by serial order.

Feel free to use this miraculous salt as a part of your daily, bath, beauty, health, DIY recipes, cleaning or gardening routine.

Please note that the recipes in this book are

Ready to get started?

Let's go!

USING EPSOM SALT FOR HEALTH

Epsom Salt can be great for your overall health. Incorporating it into your daily, weekly or fortnightly health routine is not only amazingly easy and convenient but also a safe, natural and affordable way to relieve common ailments and stimulate your body's natural immunity.

Here are some awesome Epsom Salt recipes:

USE 1: FLU RELIEF VIA EPSOM SALT

Do you want to reap the immune strengthening benefits of Epsom Salt? All you need to do is to soak yourself in this relaxing, effective and simple flu-fighting remedy.

Simply add 2 cups of Epsom Salt, 1 cup Baking soda, 5 drops of Eucalyptus essential oil, 7 drops of Tea tree essential oil, 4 drops of ginger essential oil in a tub full of warm water. Soak for at least 30 minutes.

USE 2: ANTI FLU BATH

Heard about the miraculous benefits of green tea? It is loaded with immunity strengthening anti-oxidants that enable your cells to fight off the germs which are making you sick.

List of ingredients:

1 cup Green tea (steeped for five minutes)

1 cup Epsom Salt

1 tbsp. Garlic powder

10 drops Peppermint essential oil

5 drops Lavender essential oil

A tub full of Warm water

Directions:

Add all the ingredients in the tub and soak body in bath for at least 20 minutes.

USE 3: LEMON AND EPSOM SALT BATH FOR FIGHTING COMMON COLD AND FLU

Ginger is a natural decongestant and lemon give this bath an amazing freshness.

List of ingredients:

Juice of 1 Lemon

1 cup Epsom Salt

2 inch Ginger root (powdered or very thinly sliced)

10 drops Tea tree essential oil

A tub full of Warm water

Directions:

Add all the ingredients in the tub and soak body in bath for at least 20 minutes.

USE 4: SOOTHING BATH SOAK FOR PAINS AND ACHES

This soak is extremely effective in case you are experiencing tired or fatigued muscles or even pain in joints. The Lavender essential oil used in the soak helps you beat all stress and relax.

List of ingredients:

1 cup Epsom Salt

10 drops Lavender essential oil

A tub full of Warm water

Directions:

Add all the ingredients in the tub and soak body in bath for at least 20 minutes.

USE 5: ANTI INFLAMMATORY SOAK

The combination of Chamomile and magnesium sulfate make this bath soak extremely relaxing and anti-inflammatory too.

List of ingredients:

1 cup Epsom Salt

10 drops Chamomile essential oil

10 drops Sweet Marjoram essential oil

1 tsp. Cinnamon powder

A tub full of Warm water

Directions:

Add all the ingredients in the tub and soak body in bath for at least 20 minutes.

USE 6: PMS SOOTHING SOAK

Chamomile essential oil used in combination with Epsom Salt is great to soothe symptoms of PMS.

List of ingredients:

1 cup Epsom Salt

15 drops Chamomile essential oil

A tub full of Warm water

Directions:

Add all the ingredients in the tub and soak body in bath for at least 20 minutes. Do not rinse off – just towel dry and wrap yourself in a warm blanket for at least thirty minutes after the soak.

USE 7: PAIN RELIEVING BATH SOAK

Epsom Salt has been since time immemorial to relieve aches and pains. It helps in soothing stiff muscles and becomes even more impactful when used in combination with Eucalyptus, Peppermint and Clary Sage essential oils.

List of ingredients:

1 cup Epsom Salt

10 drops Eucalyptus essential oil

5 drops Clary Sage essential oil

5 drops Peppermint essential oil

A tub full of Warm water

Directions:

Add all the ingredients in the tub and soak body in bath for at least 20 minutes.

USE 8: ANTI SPSMODIC BATH SOAK

This recipe uses Thyme and Rosemary essential oils which elevate the anti-spasmodic properties of Epsom Salt.

List of ingredients:

1 cup Epsom Salt

10 drops Thyme essential oil

10 drops Rosemary essential oil

1 tsp. Cumin powder

A tub full of Warm water

Directions:

Add all the ingredients in the tub and soak body in bath for at least 20 minutes to experience instantaneous relief from muscle spasms, back ache and stomach ache.

USE 10: ANTI ARTHRITIC BATH SOAK

This recipe uses Ginger essential oil which not only eases back pain and enhances mobility but also treats rheumatic and arthritic pains, muscle spasms and sprains.

List of ingredients:

1 cup Epsom Salt

10 drops Ginger essential oil

5 drops Lavender essential oil

1 tsp. Cinnamon powder

A tub full of Warm water

Directions:

Add all the ingredients in the tub and soak body in bath for at least 20 minutes. Repeat this every day for at least a fortnight to experience amazing arthritic relief.

USE 11: ARTHRITIC RELIEF VIA EPSOM SALT

Simply soaking your body in three cups of Epsom Salt dissolved in a tub full of warm water can help you get rid of a debilitating condition called arthritis.

This remedy is a lot cheaper than many commercially available products. You can even use it selectively. Want to help the pain in your hands? Soak in a bowl of Epsom salt infused warm water.

Use some lemon essential oil to add a dash of instant energy.

USE 12: EPSOM SALT BLOOD SUGAR CONTROLLER

Research proves that low levels of magnesium in the body have a major role to play in diabetes and insulin resistance. An occasional dose of minerals via the Epsom Salt helps in regulating the blood sugar level and improving insulin resistance. All you need to do is drink a glassful of Epsom salt infused filtered water. Add a tablespoon of Epsom Salt to one glass filtered water. Drink slowly and then drink a glass of pure, unadulterated filtered water to get rid of the after taste. Use this remedy only after consulting your medical practitioner.

USE 13: INSULIN REGULATOR

In order to help with insulin resistance, you may occasionally add a tablespoon of Epsom Salt to a cup of Peppermint tea. Drink this slowly to soothe yourself and experience long term blood sugar regulation. Once again, do not use it without the guidance of a registered medical practitioner.

USE 14: BATH TO SOOTHE NERVE PAIN AND CRAMPS

The main thing that leads to decreased nerve and muscle function is fluid retention. This can be dramatically improved through the magnesium sulfate content in Epsom salt. Soak yourself in a tub full of warm water that has 2 cups Epsom Salt, 10 drops Rosemary essential oil and 5 drops Tea tree essential oil added to it.

Doing this for at least thirty minutes every day will help in elevating nerve function. s

USE 15: NERVE STIMULATING BATH

This recipe uses Basil and Anise essential oil, both of which are nerve stimulating in nature. The effect of these oils is enhanced when used with Magnesium sulfate or Epsom Salt bath.

List of Ingredients:

1 cup Epsom Salt

10 drops Basil essential oil

5 drops Anise essential oil

A tub of warm water

Directions:

Add all the ingredients in the tub and soak body in bath for at least 20 minutes. Repeat this a few times every week.

USE 17: NERVE BALANCING BATH

The Bergamot essential oil used in this Epsom Salt bath works wonders in balancing your nervous system.

List of Ingredients:

2 cups Epsom Salt

10 drops Bergamot essential oil

5 drops Lavender essential oil

A tub of warm water

Directions:

USE 18: EPSOM SALT BATH TO RELIEVE MUSCLE STIFFNESS

Muscle stiffness can be easily relieved by mixing two cups of Epsom Salt in a tub of warm water. Add 10 drops of German Chamomile and 5 drops of Fennel oil too.

USE 19: INDIGESTION RELIEF REMEDY

Indigestion is an extremely common malady that leads to severe discomfort at times. Epsom Salt comes as a natural and handy solution in this case. A tbsp. of Epsom Salt can be dissolved in a cup of warm water to soothe an upset stomach and curb excessive acid production.

USE 20: EPSOM SALT FOR INSOMNIA

Suffering from insomnia? Epsom alt can quickly come to your rescue here. Simply add one cup of Epsom Salt to a tub full of warm water. Add a few drops of Chamomile essential oil along with 5 drops of Jasmine essential oil for added tranquility. Soak yourself in this bath for around thirty to forty minutes.

USE 21: EPSOM SALT BATH FOR A GOOD NIGHT'S SLEEP

Using Epsom Salt with essential oils derived from Valerian root can be extremely beneficial in inducing sleep. To use, just mix 1 cup Epsom Salt and 10 drops oil from the Valerian Root into a tub full of warm water. Soak for at least 40 minutes.

USE 22: EPSOM SALT TO STIMULATE BLOOD CIRCULATION

Need a relaxing blood circulation boost? Simply, take a cup of Epsom salt along with 10 drops of Rosemary essential oil, 5 drops of Eucalyptus essential oil and 4 drops of Lavender essential oil. Dissolve in a tub full of warm water and soak yourself for around 30 minutes.

Doing this every week will lead to substantial benefits.

USE 23: EPSOM SALT TO BOOST YOUR MINERAL MAGNESIUM LEVELS

If your doctor has informed you that you are deficient in magnesium, then the first thing to do is to naturally increase the quantity of magnesium in your diet. This can be done through increasing the intake of magnesium rich foods such as almonds, beans, whole grains, sesame seeds, dark chocolate, etc. Bathing twice or thrice with any Epsom Salt recipe mentioned in the book can do the trick and help you elevate your magnesium levels.

USE 24: EPSOM SALT TO RELIEVE CONSTIPATION

Drinking a tablespoon of Epsom Salt added in a glass full of filtered water can help in relieving constipation. Make sure that you are drinking it twice a day for at least one week. You may also want to add a teaspoon of honey and juice of half a lemon into your Epsom salt water.

USE 25: EPSOM SALT FOR BLOATING

Epsom salt helps in relieving gas and bloating too. Just add a teaspoon to your ginger tea and consume twice a day. Add lime to enhance the taste.

USE 26: EPSOM SALT FOR RELIEVING GASTRITIS

Chamomile herbal tea has stomach healing properties and provides relief from gas, bloating, upset stomach and cramps. Drinking 1 tsp. of Epsom Salt in a cup of Chamomile tea twice every day can help in providing sufficient relief from bloating and gas.

USE 27: EPSOM SALT FOR GOUT

Epsom salt can work wonders in gout patients due its natural uric acid flushing properties. Take a cup of Epsom salt and add in a tub full of warm water. Also add a few drops of Peppermint essential oil and Eucalyptus essential oil into this bath. Soak yourself for at least thirty minutes. Repeat every day for at least fifteen days.

USE 28: DETOXIFICATION WITH EPSOM SALT

Try and eat only veggies and fruits on the day of your detox. Quit eating or drinking by 2:00pm and prepare to consume Epsom Salt in filtered water. To make this water and Epsom Salt mixture, mix 4 tbsp. Epsom Salt in 3 cups of water. Begin drinking this mixture at around 6:00pm. Drink in regular intervals at around 6:00pm, 8:00pm, 10:00pm and then next day at 7:00am. Eat only fruits the next day too. You may experience diarrhea. Don't worry, that is your body flushing out the toxins!

USE 29: EPSOM SALT DRINK FOR RELIEVING FEVER AND HEADACHE

Soak a washcloth in a mixture of apple cider vinegar, Epsom Salt and water and place these on the forehead and tummy of the patient. You can also wrap it around the patient's feet.

USE 30: FEVER RELIEVING EPSOM SALT BATH

An Epsom Salt warm water bath sometimes brings instantaneous fever relief. Dissolve two cups of Epsom Salt in a tub of warm water. Mix one cup of Apple Cider vinegar to this water and add five drops of Cinnamon essential oil to say goodbye to fever.

FIRST AID WITH EPSOM SALT

Epsom Salt can help you relieve some of the most common first aid fiascos. From rashes to bites to stings, this little treasure can do it all.

USE 31: HEAL YOUR SUNBURNS WITH EPSOM SALT

Spraying Epsom Salt solution over your sunburns can help in fast healing. All you need is a spray bottle filled with some clean, filtered water. Dissolve one tablespoon of Epsom salt in this water along with 10 drops of Lavender essential oil and 5 drops of Rose essential oil.

USE 32: EPSOM SALT SUNBURN HEALER

Well, this is another miraculous sunburn healing recipe involving Epsom Salt and essential oils. Just add 5 drops of Lemon essential oil along with 2 heaped tablespoons of Epsom Salt into a cup of water. Dip a clean washcloth in this and apply on impacted area once every two hours.

USE 33. RELIEVE BEE STINGS WITH EPSOM SALT

Washing the impacted area with Epsom Salt solution can help in soothing bee stings.

USE 34: EPSOM SALT BATH TO HELP IN SWELLING FROM BEE STINGS

This one is simple too. Soak yourself in any of the above mentioned Epsom Salt bath for around 30 minutes and marvel at the manner in which irritation and swelling goes away.

USE 35: EPSOM SALT AND ALOE VERA STING SOOTHER

Mix a tablespoon of Epsom Salt in a cup of warm water and boil until the water reduces to half a cup. Let the mixture cool down and add two teaspoons of pure aloe vera gel. Store in the refrigerator and apply as often as required.

USE 36: EPSOM SALT BUG BITE REMEDY

This Epsom Salt solution is superbly effective and easy to whip too. Boil a cup full of water and mix 2 teaspoons of Epsom Salt into it. Continue to stir till the solution reduces to half a cup. Let it cool down and place in the refrigerator. Apply the pasty substance directly on the impacted area.

USE 37: EPSOM SALT AND LAVENDER BUG BITE RELIEVER

Dissolve 2 tablespoons of Epsom Salt along with 10 drops of Lavender essential oil in a cup of warm water. Let it cool down and apply directly on the impacted area using a clean washcloth. Do not forget to clean and dry the area first.

USE 38: EPSOM SALT BUG BITE SOOTHER

Take 2 tablespoons of Epsom Salt and dissolve in a cup of warm water. Add 10 drops of Tea tree essential oil and 5 drops of Chamomile essential oil into the mixture and apply on impacted area using a clean washcloth.

USE 39: USING EPSOM SALT FOR TROUBLESOME SPLINTERS

Spray some Epsom Salt on that troublesome splinter and tie a clean washcloth over it. Leave it overnight. Doing this for several days can help you say bye-bye to that nasty splinter.

USE 40: USING EPSOM SALT FOR WOUNDS

Mix 5 tbsp. cold water, 2 tbsp. Epsom Salt, and 10 drops Lavender essential oil. Apply this paste over the wounds and experiencing immediate healing.

USE 41: EPSOM SALT BATH FOR INFLAMED WOUNDS

This bath soak not only helps in healing the wounds but also helps in soothing the inflammation. Just mix 2 heaped tablespoons of Epsom Salt in a tubful of warm water. Add 10 drops of Geranium essential oil to this and soak yourself for around 25 minutes. Repeat it a few times in a week to experience complete healing.

USE 42: HEALING BRUISES WITH EPSOM SALT

Mix 5 tbsp. cold water, 2 tbsp. Epsom Salt, and 10 drops Lavender essential oil. Apply this paste over the wounds and experiencing immediate healing.

USE 43: EPSOM SALT BATH FOR BRUISED SKIN

The combination of Chamomile, Lavender and magnesium sulfate make this bath soak amazingly effective for bruised and inflamed skin.

List of ingredients:

1 cup Epsom Salt

10 drops Chamomile essential oil

10 drops Lavender essential oil

1 tsp. Basil powder

A tub full of Warm water

Directions:

Add all the ingredients in the tub and soak body in bath for at least 30 minutes.

USE 44: EPSOM SALT SOAK FOR THOSE NASTY HANGOVERS

Experiencing a hangover? Soaking in an Epsom salt bath can help you feel better instantaneously.

USE 45: EPSOM SALT FOR ALCOHOL TOXICITY

Alcohol toxicity is a result of and also leads to hangovers. Your best bet to detoxify your body and enable the magnesium ions restore their balance is by creating and soaking yourself into a luxurious Epsom Salt bath. To create this recipe, mix 2 cups of Epsom Salt in a tub full of warm water. Add 10 drops each of Lemon, Tea tree and Peppermint essential oils. Soak yourself for at least 45 minutes in order to stimulate your senses and clear your foggy mind.

USE 46: EPSOM SALT SOAK FOR THE HORRIBLE JET LAG

Jet is definitely not pretty! And that wear and tear of the mind and body is just so much bad – tiredness and fogginess are the last things you want to experience after landing at your destination. Soak yourself in an Epsom Salt bath for around thirty minutes to experience the best sleep you have ever had.

USE 47: EPSOM SALT FOR NAUSEA

Nausea is sometimes associated with jet lag and Epsom Salt comes in handy at this time too. Just use any one of the amazing bath recipes mentioned in the book and soak yourself for 20 minutes to get rid of the nausea and vomiting.

USE 48: POISON IVY EPSOM SALT COMPRESS

Mix 1 tbsp. Epsom Salt in 5 tbsp. of cold water. Add a few drops of Lavender essential oil into this paste and apply over the impacted area to get rid of the allergy.

USE 49: EPSOM SALT FOR THE ITCHING SKIN

It is often said that this miraculous salt can cure anything that itches or burns. Just create a cold compress using 2 tablespoons of Epsom Salt, 1 cup of cold water and 5 drops of Lavender oil. Apply on the impacted area several times a day to experience amazing relief.

USE 50: EPSOM SALT FOR DEEP CUTS

Do not apply Epsom Salt directly over the deep cuts. Instead soak yourself up in a bath created by diluting two cups of Epsom Salt in a tub full of warm water. Add some Lavender or Chamomile essential oil (not more than 5 drops) to experience added relief.

EPSOM SALT BATH RECIPES

Epsom Salt baths have a natural way of easing and relaxing the body, which helps in soothing the mind after a long tiring day. This chapter contains 25 amazing bath recipes that have been created using the miraculous Epsom Salt. Feel free to tweak these depending on the ingredients that you have handy.

USE 51: EPSOM SALT COCONUT BATH

This recipe can soothe your skin and help you unwind and relax after a long day. Dissolve 1 cup Epsom salt, 1 can of coconut milk, 10 drops of Lavender essential oil and 10 drops of Chamomile essential oil in a tub full of warm water. Soak yourself for around 30 minutes and experience ultimate miniaturization.

USE 52: MOISTURIZING EPSOM SALT BATH

List of Ingredients:

½ cup Epsom Salt

4 tbsp. olive oil

Warm water (enough to fill your tub)

10 drops Jasmine essential oil

Directions:

Dissolve all the above mentioned ingredients in your bath tub and soak yourself for 25 minutes for nice moisturizing impact.

USE 53: SATIN SMOOTH EPSOM SALT BATH

List of Ingredients:

½ cup Epsom Salt

2 tbsp. almond oil

A cap of almond milk

Warm water (enough to fill your tub)

10 drops Chamomile essential oil

Directions:

Dissolve all the above mentioned ingredients in your bath tub and soak yourself for 40 minutes to experience the best satin smooth skin ever!

USE 54: RELIEVING HEADACHE THROUGH EPSOM SALT

This is an amazing detoxifying bath recipe, which draws out toxins and balances your skin's pH level. It works wonders on migraines and headaches too. Dissolve 1 cup Epsom Salt, 1 cup Apple cider vinegar, ½ cup Baking soda, 10 drops of Chamomile essential oil and 10 drops of Peppermint essential oil in a tub full of warm water. Soak yourself for 20 minutes.

USE 55: STRESS RELIEF EPSOM SALT BATH

Dissolve 1 cup Epsom Salt, 1 cup Baking soda, ½ cup Olive oil, 7 drops Vanilla essential oil, 2 tsp. Witch Hazel, and 10 drops Lavender essential oil in a tub full of warm water. Soak yourself for thirty minutes to experience immediate stress relief and calmness.

USE 56: MIGRAINE RELIEF EPSOM SALT BATH

List of Ingredients:

2 cups Epsom Salt

Warm water (enough to fill your tub)

10 drops Eucalyptus essential oil

5 drops Rosemary essential oil

Directions:

Dissolve all the above mentioned ingredients in your bath tub and soak yourself for 20-30 minutes to experience instant relief from migraines.

USE 57: EPSOM SALT STRESS FREE BATH

The Lavender in this bath not only uplifts your mood but also provides a soothing effect. Not to mention, the headache relief from Peppermint and Rosemary essential oils.

List of Ingredients:

2 cups Epsom Salt

Warm water (enough to fill your tub)

10 drops Peppermint essential oil

5 drops Rosemary essential oil

5 drops Lavender essential oil

1 teaspoon Rose essence

Directions:

Dissolve all the above mentioned ingredients in your bath tub and soak yourself for 20-30 minutes to experience instant relief from migraines.

USE 58: EPSOM SALT BODY ACHE RELIEF BATH

List of Ingredients:

2 cups Epsom Salt

Warm water (enough to fill your tub)

10 drops Eucalyptus essential oil

5 drops Roman Chamomile essential oil

5 drops Lavender essential oil

Directions:

Dissolve all the above mentioned ingredients in your bath tub and soak yourself for around 25 minutes to experience instant relief from migraines.

USE 59: EPSOM SALT BATH TO HEAL NEURALGIA

Neuralgia can be really painful and Epsom Salt can work wonders there as well. Just mix two cups of Epsom Salt in tub full of warm water. Add 5 drops of Helichrysum essential oil and 10 drops of Peppermint essential oil to this mixture. Soak yourself for around 15 minutes. You can increase the duration to 30 minutes gradually. Also increase the quantity of Epsom Salt to 3 cups gradually. Soak yourself in this bath at least three times in a week to witness amazing results.

USE 60: EPSOM SALT BATH TO HEAL NEUROPATHY

The tingling sensation in hands and feet can sometimes worsen into Carpal Tunnel or other complications. Luckily, Epsom Salt comes as your trusted companion in this case too!

List of Ingredients:

2 cups Epsom Salt

Warm water (enough to fill your tub)

10 drops Patchouli essential oil

5 drops Tangerine essential oil

5 drops Ylang Ylang essential oil

Directions:

Dissolve all the above mentioned ingredients in your bath tub and soak yourself for around 30 minutes to experience relief from the tingling sensation. Repeat this process a few times each week.

USE 61: ESSENTIAL OIL BATH TO TREAT INSOMNIA

2 cups Epsom salt is mixed with 10 drops of roman Chamomile oil and 5 drops of Ylang Ylang oil and dissolved into a tubful of warm water. Soak yourself in this bath for 20 minutes every night to experience the most peaceful sleep ever.

USE 62: GENERAL WELL BEING BATH SALT

Dissolve 2 cups Epsom Salt, 1 cup Olive oil, 10 drops Eucalyptus oil and 10 drops Peppermint oil in a tub full of warm water and soak yourself for around 20 minutes to elevate general well-being.

USE 63: EPSOM SALT BATH TO RECLAIM YOUR SINUSES

List of Ingredients:

2 cups Epsom Salt

Warm water (enough to fill your tub)

10 drops Clove oil

2 drops Peppermint essential oil

Directions:

Dissolve all the above mentioned ingredients in your bath tub and soak yourself for around 25 minutes to clear those blocked nasal passages and relieve all respiratory inflammation.

USE 64: EPSOM OIL BATH FOR VARICOSE VEINS

A simple bath soak every day can help you get rid of varicose veins naturally. Just take 2 cups of Epsom Salt and dissolve in a tub of warm water. Soak for at least 20 minutes, preferably twice every day.

USE 65: EPSOM OIL ANTI-INFLAMMATORY AND MOISTURIZING BODY BATH

List of Ingredients:

2 cups Epsom Salt

Warm water (enough to fill your tub)

10 drops Orange oil

10 drops Helichrysum essential oil

1 cup coconut milk

2 tbsp. olive oil

Directions:

Dissolve all the above mentioned ingredients in your bath tub and soak yourself for at least 45 minutes three times in a week.

USE 66: EPSOM OIL BATH SALT FOR AGELESS SKIN

Take 2 cups of Epsom Salt and dissolve in a tub full of warm water. Dissolve 10 drops of Neroli essential oil and 5 drops of Myrrh essential oil in this water. Soak yourself for atleast 20 minutes every day to reveal fresh, wrinkle free ageless skin.

USE 67: EPSOM SALT ANTI-WRINKLE BATH

Mix 1 cup Epsom Salt with 10 drops each of Ylang Ylang, Patchouli, Tea tree and Lavender essential oil. Shake it properly and dissolve in a tub full of warm water.

Soak yourself for at least 40 minutes every alternate day.

USE 68: EPSOM SALT BATH SALT FOR HAY FEVER

Mix 2 cups of Epsom salt in a tub of warm water. Add 10 drops of Tea tree essential oil and 5 drops of Roman Chamomile essential oil to this water and soak yourself for around 15-20 minutes twice a day.

USE 69: EPSOM SALT BATH FOR CLEAR SKIN

Mix a cup of Epsom Salt with 5 drops each of Bergamot, Tea Tree and Oregano essential oil. Dissolve in a tub of warm water and soak yourself for around 40 minutes. Repeat thrice a week for amazing, clear, acne free skin.

USE 70: EPSOM SALT TO TREAT ACNE SCARS

Dissolve a cup of Epsom Salt and 5 drops each of Frankincense, Carrot seed and Lavender oil into a tub full of warm water and soak yourself up for 20 minutes each day. Doing this for fifteen to twenty days can help in completely healing the acne scars.

USE 71: EPSOM SALT FOR SKIN BRIGHTENING

A cup of Epsom Salt, 5 drops of Jasmine, Lemon and 3Lavender essential oils combined with a tub of warm water is the perfect recipe to brighten your skin. Soak every day for fifteen minutes. Visible results can be seen in 15-20 days.

USE 72: EPSOM SALT TO CURE COLD SORES

10 drops of Tea tree essential oil, 5 drops of Sage essential oil, 5 drops of Sandalwood essential oil and 1 cup of Epsom Salt dissolved in a tub of warm water can help in curing cold sores.

USE 73: EPSOM SALT BATH FOR MOOD SWINGS

This one is extremely effective in PMS, depression and other mood swings. Immerse yourself in the luxury of Epsom Salt bath created by dissolving 2 cups Epsom Salt in 1 tub full of warm water with 10 drops of Rose Otto essential oil and 5 drops of Jasmine essential oil.

USE 74: ENERGIZING EPSOM SALT BATH BLEND

List of Ingredients:

2 cups Epsom Salt

Warm water (enough to fill your tub)

10 drops Orange oil

10 drops Lemon essential oil

5 drops Bergamot essential oil

Directions:

Dissolve all the above mentioned ingredients in your bath tub and soak yourself for at least 20 minutes to regain the lost energy.

USE 75: ANXIETY RELIEF EPSOM SALT BATH BLEND

Mix 10 drops of Lavender essential oil, 5 drops of Clary Sage essential and 2 cups Epsom Salt in a tub full of warm water. Soak yourself in this water for 20 minutes to experience relief from anxiety and depression.

BEAUTY BENEFITS OF EPSOM SALT

The Epsom Salt beauty recipes mentioned in this chapter will ensure that your exterior is as healthful as your interior.

USE 76: EPSOM SALT EXFOLIATING SCRUB

Prepare your very own exfoliating scrub using 2 cups Epsom Salt, 4 tbsp. olive oil, juice of one medium sized lemon, 1 tbsp. basil leaf powder and 1 tbsp. oatmeal powder. Use this one of twice a week dry or in shower.

USE 77: EPSOM SALT SKIN SOOTHING SCRUB

This is prepared by mixing 1 cup Epsom Salt, 2 tbsp. Almond oil, juice of half medium sized lemon and a handful of dried rosemary leaves. Use twice a week for best results.

USE 78: EPSOM SALT ANTI ACNE SCRUB

To prepare this, mix 1 cup of Epsom Salt with 3 tbsp. of coconut oil and 5 drops of Carrot Seed oil. Use every day to notice visible reduction in acne and scars.

USE 79: EPSOM SALT SCRUB FOR FAIRNESS.

A simple Epsom Salt fairness scrub can be made by mixing a cup of Epsom Salt with 10 drops of Lemon essential oil and a tbsp. Almond oil. You must use it every day to notice visible results within 10-15 days.

USE 80: EPSOM SALT ANTI-WRINKLE SCRUB

To prepare this, mix a cup of Epsom Salt with two tablespoons of sweet almond oil and 10 drops of Frankincense essential oil. Use in shower every day.

USE 81: EPSOM SALT FACIAL CLEANSER

Mix Epsom Salt with a pinch of cinnamon and a tbsp. of coconut oil. Use it as a purifying natural cleanser.

USE 82: EPSOM SALT BASED BODY BUTTER

Mix 1 cup of Epsom Salt with 2 tbsp. of boiling water. Combine 2 tbsp. beeswax, 3 tbsp. of Shea butter, ¼ cup of olive oil and ½ cup of sweet almond oil in a jar and place this jar in a pan with water. Place this pan over medium heat and wait until the mixture melts. Blend the oil mixture and slowly add the Epsom salt mix. Now, place in the fridge to get the consistency of body butter. Apply as and when required.

USE 83: EPSOM SALT SATIN SMOOTH BODY BUTTER

Mix 1 cup of Epsom Salt with 2 tbsp. of boiling water. Combine 2 tbsp. beeswax, 3 tbsp. of Cocoa butter and ½ cup of almond oil in a jar and place this jar in a pan with water. Place this pan over medium heat and wait until the mixture melts. Blend the oil mixture and slowly add the Epsom salt mix. Now, place in the fridge to get the consistency of body butter. Apply as and when required.

USE 84: ANTI BLEMISH BODY BUTTER USING EPSOM SALT

Mix 1 cup of Epsom Salt with 2 tbsp. of boiling water. Combine 2 tbsp. beeswax, 3 tbsp. of Shea butter, ½ cup of almond oil, 20 drops of Lemon essential oil, 10 drops of Frankincense essential oil and ¼ cup of coconut oil in a jar and place this jar in a pan with water. Place this pan over medium heat and wait until the mixture melts. Blend the oil mixture and slowly add the Epsom salt mix. Now, place in the fridge to get the consistency of body butter. Apply as and when required.

USE 85: VITAMIN E RICH EPSOM SALT BODY BUTTER

This body butter is offer amazing benefits of vitamin E along with the mineral magnesium. Mix 1 cup of Epsom

Salt with 2 tbsp. of boiling water. Combine 1 cup cocoa butter and 1 cup extra virgin olive oil a jar and place this jar in a pan with water. Place this pan over medium heat and wait until the mixture melts. Now, puncture 6 capsules of vitamin E and add to the blend. Next, add the Epsom salt mix. Now, place in the fridge to get the consistency of body butter. Apply as frequently as required.

USE 86: EPSOM SALT BODY BRONZING BODY BUTTER

Nutmeg, cinnamon and cacao powder — whipped together along with Epsom Salt into a luxuriously aromatic creamy spread – wow! What a treat! To prepare, gently melt 1 cup Shea butter in a pan using the double boiler method. Next, pour 1 cup coconut oil into this and continue to stir until blended. Let the mixture cool down and add ¼ cup of almond oil, 1 tbsp. ground nutmeg, 1 tbsp. ground cinnamon and 1 tbsp. cacao powder into the mixture. Now, add 1 cup of Epsom Salt and place this mixture in the refrigerator. Whip it after 20 minutes and use as frequently as desired.

USE 87: DOUBLE MAGNESIUM MAGIC BODY BUTTER

Take ½ cup magnesium flakes in a container and pour around ½ cup of boiling water over them. Keep stirring until they are completely dissolved and a thick liquid is formed. Add 1 cup Epsom Salt to this mixture and set aside to cool.

Now, take 1 cup Shea butter, 4 tbsp. beeswax and 1 cup coconut oil in a separate pan and mix these using the double boiler method. Add the magnesium mixture and let it cool. Allow it to set in the refrigerator.

USE 88: SUPER LUSCIOUS AND NOURISHING EPSOM SALT BODY BUTTER

This one is prepared using 1 cup Epsom Salt, 1 cup Shea butter, 1 cup coconut oil, 4 tbsp. Jojoba oil and 20 drops of Rose essential oil.

Truly magical and divine!

USE 89: BYE BYE TO BLEMISHES WITH EPSOM SALT

Boil a cup of water and add 3 drops iodine along with 10 drops of Rose essential oil, 5 drops of Lavender essential oil and 1 tbsp. of Epsom Salt into it. Stir till mixed well. Allow to cool and pack in an airtight container to be stored in the refrigerator. Apply frequently over blemishes. Keep for fifteen minutes and wash with cold water.

USE 90: EPSOM SALT ANTI MARKS OINTMENT

Boil a cup of water and add a few basil leaves into it along with 1 tbsp. of Epsom Salt. Continue to stir till mixed well and until the water reduces to half a cup. Allow to cool and pack in an airtight container to be stored in the refrigerator. Use a cotton swab to apply over blemishes, let it sit for 10 minutes and rinse off with cold water.

USE 91: EPSOM SALT ANTI BLACKHEADS OINTMENT

A cup of Epsom Salt is added to 2 cups of water and boiled until a pasty consistency is achieved. 2 tbsp. of cucumber juice is added to this along with 10 drops of Lemon essential oil. This can be stored in the refrigerator and used thrice a day for visible results.

USE 92: EPSOM SALT DARK CIRCLES OINTMENT

Boil a cup of water and add 2 tbsp. Epsom Salt into it. Next, add some lemon juice and 5 drops of lime essential oil into this. Store it in an airtight container once it cools down and apply as frequently as you would like.

USE 93: EPSOM SALT OINTMENT FOR DRY AND FLAKY SKIN

Boil a cup of water and add a 2 tbsp. olive oil into it along with 1 tbsp. of Epsom Salt. Continue to stir till mixed well and until the water reduces to half a cup. Add 2 tbsp. coconut milk to this mixture and allow it to cool. Pack in an airtight container and store in the refrigerator. Use a cotton swab to apply over dry skin, let it sit for 10 minutes and rinse off with cold water.

USE 94: EPSOM SALT OINTMENT FOR PUFFY EYES

Boil a cup of water and add a 2 tbsp. extra virgin coconut oil into it along with 1 tbsp. of Epsom Salt. Continue to stir till mixed well and until the water reduces to half a cup. Add 2 tbsp. of cucumber juice to this mixture and allow it to cool. Pack in an airtight container and store in the refrigerator. Use a cotton swab to apply under the eye area, let it sit for 10 minutes and rinse off with cold water.

USE 95: EPSOM SALT OINTMENT FOR WRINKLED HANDS

Boil a cup of water and add a 2 tbsp. of sweet almond oil into it along with 1 tbsp. of Epsom Salt. Continue to stir till mixed well and until the water reduces to half a cup. Add ½ cup of coconut milk to this mixture and allow it to cool. Pack in an airtight container and store in the refrigerator. Use it as often as possible to nourish your hands.

USE 96: EPSOM SALT SCRUB FOR CHAPPED LIPS

This is an extremely simple recipe that helps in getting rid of dry, flaky, unsightly lips. Combine a teaspoon of maple syrup, 10 drops rose essential oil and a tablespoon of Epsom Salt. Apply over your dry lips to experience immediate moisture and glow!

USE 97: EPSOM SALT SCRUB FOR DRY HEELS

Get an instant pedicure at home using Epsom Salt. Dip your feet in a tub of warm water mixed with 1 tbsp. Epsom Salt. Pat dry using a towel and apply the Epsom salt ointments for wrinkled hands (recipe above) over the heels too!

USE 98: EPSOM SALT FOR ORAL HYGIENE

Gargle with a tablespoon of Epsom Salt added in a cup of warm water. Add a dash of lemon juice for flavor.

USE 99: EPSOM SALT RINSE FOR ORAL ULCERS

Oral ulcers can be extremely painful. Use 2 tbsp. Epsom Salt dissolved in a cup of room temperature water infused with a tbsp. of basil leaves to experience relief from oral ulcers.

USE 100: EPSOM SALT RISE TO PURIFY THE SCALP

Combine 2 tbsp. Epsom Salt, 1 cup hot water and ½ cup lemon juice. Allow it to cool for some time and apply to dampened scalp. Let it soak for around 10 minutes. Rinse thoroughly followed by your regular shampoo routine.

USE 101: EPSOM SALT HAIR MASK

Combine 1 cup Epsom Salt, 1 cup warm water, ½ cup lemon juice, 3 tbsp. coconut oil and 10 drops of Jasmine essential oil. Allow it to cool and apply over dampened scalp. Leave on for thirty minutes and rinse with your regular shampoo.

USE 102: EPSOM SALT NATURAL HAIR CONDITIONER

Combine 2 tbsp. sweet almond oil with 2 tbsp. Epsom Salt and 1 tbsp. baking soda. Apply like your regular conditioner and notice results within a few weeks.

USE 103: EPSOM SALT VOLUMIZING CONDITIONER

Combine 2 tbsp. Epsom Salt with 2 tbsp. Extra virgin coconut oil and use like your regular conditioner. Noticeable results will be visible in a few weeks.

USE 104: EPSOM SALT FOOT SOAK

Combine 1 cup Epsom Salt, 1 foot tub of warm water, 2 tbsp. lemon juice, ½ cup Apple cider vinegar and few drops of Lavender essential oil. Soak feet for at least thirty minutes. Repeat few times in a week.

USE 105: EPSOM SALT EYE COMPRESS

Mix 3 tbsp. Epsom Salt in 3 tbsp. hot water. Let the mixture cool down and then add some cucumber juice into it. Dip a clean washcloth and place over closed eyes for a few minutes. Repeat morning and evening for best results. !

USE 106: EPSOM SALT INFUSED SHAMPOO

Craving for extra nourishment for your hair? Mix 1 tbsp. Epsom Salt into your regular shampoo to witness some amazing nourishment and deep cleansing.

USE 107: EPSOM SALT FACE MASK FOR ACNE PRONE SKIN

Mix 1 tbsp. honey, 1 tbsp. Epsom Salt, 1 tsp. baking soda and juice of half a lemon to prepare the best face mask to treat your acne.

USE 108: EPSOM SALT FACE MASK FOR BEAUTIFUL SKIN

Mix a tablespoon of Epsom Salt with 1 tablespoon of Apple cider vinegar and ½ tablespoon honey. Apply on face, keep for 20 minutes and rinse.

USE 109: EPSOM SALT MASK FOR DRY SKIN

Blend 1 cup grated carrot, 1 cup Epsom Salt and 1 cup mayonnaise. Spread over damp skin, wait for ten minutes and remove.

USE 110: EPSOM SALT MASK FOR OILY SKIN

Blend 1 egg, 2 tbsp. Epsom Salt, 1 tbsp. non-fat dry milk and juice of 1 lemon. Apply to damp skin, wait for five minutes and rinse off.

USE 111: EPSOM SALT HAIRSPRAY REMOVER

Take a gallon of water and add one cup of Epsom Salt into it. Also add 1 cup lemon juice and let this mixture infuse overnight. The next morning, apply prior to your shampoo ritual and notice the hairspray gone!

USE 112: EPSOM SALT WHITENING TOOTHPASTE

Mix 1 tbsp. Epsom Salt with a little hydrogen peroxide. Brush your teeth with this mixture. Although it tastes terrible, it promises amazing benefits.

USING EPSOM SALT FOR WEIGHT LOSS

Bathing in a warm Epsom Salt soak helps in flushing out the toxins, which in turn leads to weight loss.

USE 113: EPSOM SALT SCRUB TO TREAT CELLULITE

Mix 4 tbsp. Honey, 2 tbsp. Epsom Salt, 2 tbsp. Brown Sugar and 1 tbsp. lemon juice. Massage into the problems areas, leave for two minutes and rinse with warm water.

USE 114: EPSOM SALT SOAK FOR RAPID WEIGHT LOSS

Add 1 cup Epsom Salt, 1 cup Apple cider vinegar, 1 tbsp. ginger powder, and 10 drops grapefruit essential oil into a tubful of warm water. Soak for 20 minutes.

USE 115: 'FIT INTO SKINNY JEANS' EPSOM SALT SOAK

Want a temporary and quick fix 'fit into the skinny jeans' remedy? Just soak yourself into a warm water tub infused with 2 cups of Epsom Salt for around 10 minutes. You will be pleasantly surprised by the instant results.

USE 120: SPECIAL EPSOM SALT RAPID WEIGHT LOSS BATH

Mix 2 cups Epsom Salt and 1 cup Baking soda into a tub full of warm water. Soak yourself in this bath for at least 25 minutes every day. If you cannot do every day, try every alternate day in order to achieve consistent and visible weight loss.

USE 121: EPSOM SALT AND ACV WEIGHT LOSS BATH

Epsom Salt and ACV can work wonders for your weight loss when used together. Dissolve 1 cup Epsom Salt and 1 cup ACV in a tub full of warm water. Soak yourself for 20 minutes every day to experience some amazing long term inch loss.

USE 122: EPSOM SALT ANTI BLOATING BATH

Add 1 cup Epsom Salt, 1 tbsp. dried ginger and 10 drops of Eucalyptus essential oil into a tub full of warm water. Soak yourself for at least 20 minutes three times a week.

USE 123: EPSOM SALT WEIGHT LOSS DRINK

Mix 1 tbsp. Epsom Salt and 1 gm. Cumin powder into a glass of warm water. Drink slowly followed by another glass of normal, filtered water. Visible results can be seen in thirty days or less.

USE 124: EPSOM SALT WEIGHT LOSS AID

You can create your own mild Epsom Salt induced water by mixing 1 tbsp. Epsom Salt in 1 liter of water. Sip throughout the day.

USE 125: EPSOM SALT ANTI BLOATING DRINK

Mix 1 tbsp. Epsom Salt, 1 tsp. grated ginger and 1 tsp. ACV in a glass full of water. Drink slowly for three consecutive days. Give a gap of three days and drink again for three days. Continue this for as long as you can.

EPSOM SALT TO NOURISH YOUR GARDEN

Just as Epsom Salt is great for the body and mind, it can work wonders for nourishing your plants too.

USE 126: EPSOM SALT AS FERTILIZER

Dilute 5 tbsp. Epsom Salt per 1 gallon of water. Allow the mixture to dissolve and transfer into a spray bottle. Spritz directly on to your plants once per month in replacement of regular watering.

USE 127: HEALTHY PEPPERS, TOMATOES AND ROSES

Mix 1 tbsp. Epsom Salt in a gallon of water. Spray on surrounding soil every few weeks.

USE 128: EPSOM SALT DIRECT APPLICATION FOR TOMATOES AND PEPPERS

Mix 2 tbsp. Epsom Salt in half a bucket of water. Scoop a small handful and sprinkle it at the base of your plants.

USE 129: EPSOM SALT INSECT AND PEST REPELLANT

Just put some Epsom salt into areas frequented by pests and get pleasantly surprised with the amazing difference.

USE 130: EPSOM SALT FERTILIZER FOR FRUIT TREES

Mixing Epsom Salt in the soil near your fruits will do the trick here.

USE 131: EPSOM SALT SPRAY FOR GREENER GRASS

Spray Epsom Salt over your grass every three months and experience the best lawns ever.

USE 132: LUSCIOUS LAWNS USING EPSOM SALT

You can even combine Epsom salt with water and spray over your grass. I bet, you will be amazed at the quality of your lawns.

USE 133: EPSOM SALT TO DEODORIZE COMPOST

Just add some Epsom Salt into your compost and experience complete deodorization.

USE 134: EPSOM SALT TO REMOVE STUMPS

Epsom Salt can be poured over stumps to remove them too.

USE 135: EPSOM SALT FOR BETTER FLOWERING

Addition of Epsom Salt into the garden can help in better flowering.

USE 136: EPSOM SALT FOR BETTER NUTRIENT ABSORPTION

Addition of Epsom Salt into the soil can help plants take up vital nutrients, eliminating the need for chemical fertilizers.

USE 137: EPSOM SAT TO PREVENT LEAF CURLING

Application of Epsom Salt near the base of leaves will prevent them from curling.

USE 138: EPSOM SALT TO COUNTER TRANSPLANT SHOCK

Roots can be damaged and transplant shock can occur when you move plants from one place to another. After planting, water the plants with 1 gallon of water mixed with 1 tbsp. Epsom Salt.

USE 139: EPSOM SALT FOR PALM TREES FRIZZLE TOP

Magnesium deficiency in palms can lead to frizzle tops. Apply Epsom Salt around the base and drench the leaves and crown with a liquid mixture of 1 tbsp. to 1 gallon of water.

USE 140: EPSOM SALT WEED KILLER

Mix 2 cups Epsom Salt with 1 gallon of vinegar. Add a liquid dish soap into the mixture and put in a spray bottle. Then spray over weeds, carefully avoiding leaves and other plants. This will kill the weeds in the most efficient way.

EPSOM SALT FOR HOUSEHOLD USE

Finally, it is time to discover the wonderful uses of Epsom Salt in your home.

USE 141: EPSOM SALT CLEANER FOR TILES

Combine 1 cup Epsom Salt, 1 cup baking soda and ½ cup vinegar. Scrub over tiles using clockwise motion. Rinse thoroughly.

USE 142: POT AND PAN CLEANER

You can clean your pots and pans with Epsom salt too.

USE 143: EPSOM SALT HOUSE PLANT REFRESHER

Spraying Epsom Salt over house plants can help in maintenance.

USE 144: EPSOM SALT CARPET CLEANER

A mixture of Epsom Salt and water works well when it comes to cleaning carpets and rugs.

USE 145: EPSOM SALT RUST REMOVERS

A combination of Epsom Salt, water and lemon juice can be used to scrub off the rust.

USE 146: EPSOM SALT FABRIC SOFTENER

Add ½ tablespoon Epsom Salt and 10 drops of Jasmine essential oil to your favorite laundry cleaner and drool over the softness of your clothes.

USE 147: EPSOM SALT TO FILL HOLES IN THE WALL

A thick paste of Epsom Salt can help in filling the holes in the wall.

USE 148: EPSOM SALT WASHING MACHINE CLEANSER

A mixture of Epsom Salt and white vinegar can be used to clean washing machines too.

USE 149: REGENERATING YOUR CAR BATTERY

Dissolve about an ounce of Epsom Salt in warm water and add to each battery cell.

USE 150: FROST YOUR WINDOWS FOR CHRISTMAS

Dreaming of a white Christmas and the weather doesn't seem to cooperate? Well, Epsom salt can come to your rescue here too. Mix Epsom Salt with stale bear until it stops dissolving. Apply this mixture to your windows with a sponge. The windows look frosted once the mixture dries.

CONCLUSION

You have now discovered the numerous ways Epsom Salt can be incorporated into your daily life and routine. Thank you for purchasing this book and joining me in the journey to explore and incorporate natural and effective ingredients for a variety of everyday tasks. I hope that you will found these tips, and recipes to be useful for your health and home. Wishing you much success.